YOUR KNOWLEDGE HAS VALUE

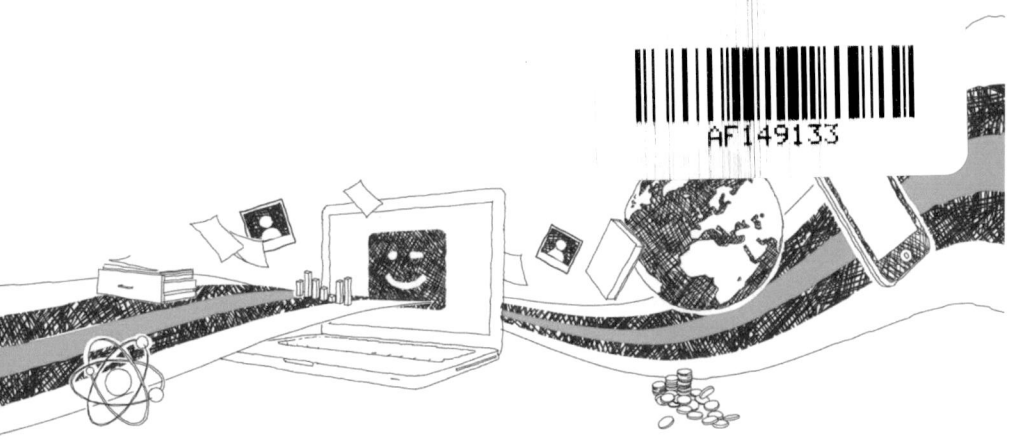

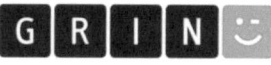

Bibliographic information published by the German National Library:

The German National Library lists this publication in the National Bibliography; detailed bibliographic data are available on the Internet at http://dnb.dnb.de .

Imprint:

Copyright © 2017 GRIN Verlag, Open Publishing GmbH
Print and binding: Books on Demand GmbH, Norderstedt Germany
ISBN: 9783668590823

This book at GRIN:

http://www.grin.com/en/e-book/383553/sleep-disorders-a-short-overview

Patrick Kimuyu

Sleep Disorders. A short Overview

GRIN Publishing

GRIN - Your knowledge has value

Since its foundation in 1998, GRIN has specialized in publishing academic texts by students, college teachers and other academics as e-book and printed book. The website www.grin.com is an ideal platform for presenting term papers, final papers, scientific essays, dissertations and specialist books.

Visit us on the internet:

http://www.grin.com/

http://www.facebook.com/grincom

http://www.twitter.com/grin_com

Sleep Disorders

Patrick Kimuyu

Abstract

Sleep plays significant health and physical roles in the body because it is linked to the humoral responses. As such, the quality of sleep acts as an indicator of one's optimal health and physical well-being. However, the quality of sleep is usually interfered with by sleep disorders. Sleep disorders interrupt sleep by causing sleep disturbances. The most common sleep disorders are insomnia, sleep apnea, narcolepsy, restless leg syndrome and circadian rhythm problems.

Due to the biological mechanisms involved in sleep disorders, this paper will discuss sleep disorders and explain the role of hormones in sleep deprivation.

Introduction

Sleep has been found to play fundamental biological roles in humans. It is linked to emotional well-being and physical health. This is why sleep deprivation leads to numerous consequences including reduced job performance, accidents, poor health, and stress episodes. From a biological perspective, sleep can be used as an indicator of good health because sleeping tendencies change with an individual's health. For instance, a good sleep is associated with optimal health and wellness; whereas sleeping problems are associated to a health problem. In most cases, persistent sleeping problems have been identified to be significant indicators of underlying mental health or medical problems (Carskadon & Dement, 2000). In practice, the impacts of sleep in an individual's health can be explained by the changes experienced after sleep deprivation, even under minimal situations. Sleep deprivation has been found to influence an individual's mood, ability to respond to stress, efficacy, and energy generation for physical activities in daily life. It is worth noting that loss of sleep in some occasions is caused by internal factors such as stress or external factors including changes of abiotic factors in the ecosystem such as climatic conditions. However, when sleeping problems occur repeatedly leading an interference with an individual's daily life, it might be an indication that one is suffering from a sleep disorder (Guilleminault, 2005). This phenomenon is attributable to changes in the endocrine system leading to hormonal imbalances. This explains why most women begin experiencing sleep disorders during menopause due a decrease in estrogen and progesterone levels. This indicates how the endocrine system influences sleep in humans. Therefore, this paper will give a comprehensive overview on sleep disorders and explain the role of hormones in sleep deprivation.

Common Sleep Disorders

Currently, a number of sleep disorders have been identified although some sleep disorders are interrelated; the occurrence a certain sleep disorder leads to the occurrence of another disorder. Some of the most common sleep disorders are insomnia, narcolepsy, restless legs syndrome, sleep apnea, and the circadian rhythm disorders.

Insomnia

Insomnia, which is characterized by trouble staying asleep or falling asleep, is regarded as the most common sleep disorder (Parmer, 2006). In reality, most sleep complaints are related insomnia and it is usually defined by the quality of sleep, but not necessarily the hours spend in a sleep. Ideally, sleep is meant to create rest of the body, biological phenomenon that occurs under low metabolic rates in the body and cardiac rhythm. Therefore, the indented outcome of this biological phenomenon is feeling refreshed after sleep. However, insomnia is defined as the lack of the intended outcomes. Ordinarily, insomnia can be short-term or chronic depending on the primary causes of the condition. Insomnia can be caused by a single factor such as stress or a collection of conditions.

Despite the diversity of factors that cause insomnia, an array of signs and symptoms has been identified. In most cases, insomnia in manifested by difficulty staying asleep during the night or falling asleep. It is also characterized by exhaustion after sleep or light and fragmented sleep sessions. Other symptoms associated with insomnia are fatigue, lack of concentration in daily activities and daytime drowsiness. Dependency on alcohol or sleeping pills due to problems falling asleep is also considered as an implication of insomnia (Smith, Saisan, Robinson & Segal, 2015[b]).

It is reported that insomnia is commonly caused by persistent stress, inactive lifestyle, anxiety or depression disorders, shift work, alcohol consumption, relationship problems, and stimulants such as cocaine and caffeine. In addition, environmental factors have also been found to cause insomnia. For instance, noisy environment or changes in lighting have been found to cause transient episodes of insomnia which subside upon withdrawal of the environmental triggers. Insomnia is also caused by other sleep disorders or health problems (Parmer, 2006). For instance, psychological conditions such as post-traumatic stress disorder and bipolar disorder have been found to be some of the psychological conditions that lead to the occurrence of insomnia. On the other hand, insomnia can be caused by some medical conditions. Some of the medical conditions that have been found to cause insomnia include kidney disease, acid reflux, chronic pain, hyperthyroidism, and cancer. Other medical conditions that are believed to cause insomnia are Parkinson's disease, allergies and asthma. It is also worth noting that some medications cause insomnia. For instance, medications for high blood pressure; antidepressants; diuretics; thyroid hormone; corticosteroids; and pain relievers such as Excedrin and Midol, which contain caffeine, are known to cause insomnia.

Moreover, insomnia is caused by other sleep disorders including sleep apnea, restless legs syndrome and narcolepsy (Smith, Saisan, Robinson & Segal, 2015[a]).

Sleep Apnea

Sleep apnea is the second sleep disorder that cause sleep deprivation in people. Sleep apnea is considered as life-threatening disorder because it interferes with breathing volumes. In sleep apnea, breathing is interrupted by airway blockages. As a result, people suffering from sleep apnea experience awakenings during sleep; thus affecting the quality of sleep. However, this condition is difficult to identify because most people who have awakenings due to sleep apnea do not notice.

Ordinarily, sleep apnea is characterized by a number of signs and symptoms. Some of these symptoms include exhaustion after sleep, depression, chronic snoring, and snorting during sleep. It is also characterized by dry throat, nasal congestion, shortness of breath, headaches, and chest pain (Smith, Saisan, Robinson & Segal, 2015[b]). In some cases, people suffering from sleep apnea experience drowsiness during the day with some decrease physical activity. On the other hand, causes of sleep apnea include the abnormal contraction and relaxation of throat muscles, large tonsils, bony structure of the head and neck, as well as the formation of soft fat tissue in the windpipe, a condition commonly experienced under overweight conditions (NIH, 2012).

Narcolepsy

Narcolepsy is a sleep disorder that causes excessive daytime sleepiness. This disorder has been found to be caused by the dysfunction of the brain centers involved in sleep regulation. Ordinarily, people suffering from this disorder experience sleep attacks during their daily activities such as working, conversation or driving in which brain mechanisms to maintain alertness fails leading to an unexpected falling asleep.

Narcolepsy is usually characterized by muscle weakness during episodes of strong emotions such as anger and laughing. In addition, intense dreaming shortly after falling asleep and numbness of the limbs in the morning are considered as some of the most principle signs and symptoms of narcolepsy. Moreover, hallucinations, hearing strange things before falling into deep sleep, are a characteristic of narcolepsy (Smith, Saisan, Robinson & Segal, 2015[b]).

4

Restless Legs Syndrome

Restless legs syndrome is the fourth form of sleep disorder, and it is characterized by frequent movement of legs while sleeping. People suffering from this disorder experience a strong urge for moving their legs during rest owing to uncomfortable, creeping or tingling sensations which are responsible for the restlessness of the legs. In addition, restless legs syndrome is manifested by repetitive jerking or cramping of legs, especially at night when one is asleep.

Circadian Rhythms-associated Disorders

There are other sleep problems that involve the circadian rhythms. Some of these disorders include delayed sleep phase disorder, jet lag and shift work sleeping disorders. These circadian rhythm disorders are caused by interruptions in circadian rhythms. They occur due changes in hormonal imbalances especially those involved in sleep regulation such as melatonin, thyroid hormone, growth hormone and cortisol (Krueger et al., 1998). For instance, delayed sleep phase disorder occurs when someone feels sleep too late in the evening and wakes up late the following morning. In this case, the 24-hour sleep-and-wake cycle in not regulated normally by environmental triggers, primarily light changes. On the other hand, work shift sleep disorder occurs due to conditioned reflex in which people who alternate day and night work shifts experienced unsynchronized sleep cycles. Similarly, jet lag sleep disorder occurs due to changes in ecological factors. It occurs mostly to people who travel by plane across different time zones (Smith, Saisan, Robinson & Segal, 2015[b]).

Endocrine System and Sleep Disorders

Despite the specific causes of sleep disorders which are either physical or psychological in nature, the endocrine system exerts the ultimate influence that can be used to explain the pathophysiology of these disorders. From a biological perspective, hormones play significant roles in sleep deprivation, the principle characteristic of all sleep disorders (Guilleminault, 2005). Therefore, an understanding on the role of humoral system in sleep deprivation serves as the principle approach in the treatment of sleep disorders.

Thyroid Hormone

Under sleep deprivation, thyroid hormone is believed to be responsible for sleep deprivation physiology. According to Pereira & Andersen (2014), the pituitary gland increases its release of thyroid stimulating hormone leading to the increase of thyroid hormone production. This phenomenon is associated to changes in the neural circuits. Therefore, thyroid axis is believed to be responsible for sleep deprivation, although the mechanism is not well understood.

Cortisol

Cortisol has been found to play principal roles in sleep regulation. Ordinarily, cortisol levels changes with environmental triggers; reaching its peak at 9.00 AM in the morning and falling significantly towards the midnight. Bush & Hudson (2010), cortisol is linked to the circadian rhythms during sleep. It is reported that sleep triggers cortisol release leading to a significant increase in cortisol levels in blood within the first stage of sleep, 2-3 hours (Buckley & Schatzberg, 2005). In the following morning, cortisol levels approaches the peak. After the peak in the mid-morning, cortisol levels are observed to exhibit gradual decline during the day until nadir (Bush & Hudson, 2010). Therefore, it is apparent that high cortisol levels in blood induce sleep; whereas low levels favor alertness. Under some sleep disorders, especially those which involve depression and anxiety as some of the major causes such as insomnia and apnea. Cortisol is responsible for daytime drowsiness because these psychological factors trigger increase in cortisol levels. This is the reason why cortisol is classified as one of the 'stress hormones.'

Melatonin

Melatonin has also been found to influence the quality of sleep. However, it is worth noting that melatonin does not regulate sleep, but its levels are influenced by sleep. During sleep deprivation, serum levels of melatonin have been found to be low. In contrast, quality sleep is characterized by high serum levels of melatonin. This hormone is really important in understanding the management of sleep disorders, in order to prevent adverse health consequences related to sleep deprivation. Melatonin is an anti-oxidant which is released from the pineal gland, and its function is removing active radicals from the body. As such, sleep deprivation may lead to the onset of diseases which are caused by active radicals such as cancer. It is also believed to play key roles in cognitive activities. Ordinarily, melatonin is known to offer protection to neurons against oxidative stress. Therefore, the high levels of oxidative stress that occurs during sleep deprivation lead to impairment of the cognitive functioning of the brain (Zhanq et al., 2013). This is why lack of melatonin has been associated with memory loss, dementia and other cognitive related disorders.

Treatment of Sleep Disorders

Regarding treatment, sleep disorders require treatment and management, more or less the same as any other disease. For instance, management requires eliminating the causes to alleviate the associated symptoms. Short-term insomnia is addressed by lifestyle changes such as avoiding caffeine, alcohol, as well as medicines that are known to disrupt sleep. It is also managed by adopting healthy bedtime habits such as relaxing before sleeping and engaging in physical exercise some few hours before bed. On the other hand, chronic insomnia, apnea, as well as all the other sleep disorders can be treated by reducing stress and anxiety triggers through Cognitive-Behavioral Therapy. In addition, medicines such as melatonin, valerian and antihistamines can help to solve sleep problems (NIH, 2011).

Conclusion

In a brief conclusion, sleep disorders are quite common, even though most people do not notice. These are disorders that deprive an individual of sleep leading to health and psychological consequences. It is apparent that sleep plays significant roles in the health and physical well-being of a person. Therefore, quality sleep is essential for a healthy living. Despite the benefits that are reaped from sleep, most people hardly get adequate sleep due to both intrinsic and external stressors. These lead to the occurrence of a sleep disorder. Some of the most common sleep disorders include insomnia, restless legs syndrome, sleep apnea, narcolepsy, and circadian rhythm sleep problems. Most of these disorders are caused by inactive lifestyle, psychological disorders, anxiety and medical conditions, and their treatment involves lifestyle changes, medication and Cognitive-Behavioral Therapy.

However, the endocrine system is believed to play key roles in influencing the signs and symptoms associated with sleep disorders. For instance, cortisol, thyroid hormone and other steroid hormones regulate sleep. In addition, the biological processes triggered by sleep deprivation such as oxidative stress require attention in order to prevent the occurrence of stress related diseases.

References

Buckley, T., & Schatzberg, Z., (2005). On The Interactions of the Hypothalamic-Pituitaryadrenal (HPA) Axis and Sleep: Normal HPA Axis Activity and Circadian Rhythm, Exemplary Sleep Disorders. *J Clin Endocrinol Metab.*, *90*(5), 3106-3114.

Bush, B., & Hudson, T., (2010). The Role of Cortisol in Sleep. *Natural Medicine Journal, 2*(6). Retrieved from http://naturalmedicinejournal.com/journal/2010-06/role-cortisol-sleep

Carskadon, M., & Dement, W., (2000). *Normal Human Sleep: An Overview. In: Kdryger, M., Dement, W., Eds. Principles and Practice of Sleep Medicine.* Philadelphia, PA: Saunders.

Guilleminault, C., (2005). Clinical Neurophysiology of Sleep Disorders: Volume 6 of Handbook of clinical neurophysiology. Amsterdam, Netherlands: Elsevier Health Sciences.

Krueger, J. M., et al., (1998). Humoral Regulation of Sleep. *Physiology, 13*(4), 189-194.

NIH (2011). *How Is Insomnia Treated?* Retrieved from https://www.nhlbi.nih.gov/health/health-topics/topics/inso/treatment

NIH (2012). *What Causes Sleep Apnea?* Retrieved from http://www.nhlbi.nih.gov/health/health-topics/topics/sleepapnea/causes

Parmer, S., (2006). Insomnia. *JAMA, 295*(24), 2952.

Pereira, J. C., & Andersen, M. L., (2014). The Role of Thyroid Hormone in Sleep Deprivation. *Med. Hypotheses, 82*(3), 350-5.

Smith, M., Saisan, J., Robinson, L., & Segal, R., (2015[a]). *Can't Sleep? Causes, Cures, and Treatments for Insomnia.* Harvard, MA: Harvard Health Publications.

Smith, M., Saisan, J., Robinson, L., & Segal, R., (2015[b]). *Sleep Disorders and Sleeping Problems.* Harvard, MA: Harvard Health Publications.

Zhanq, L., et al., (2013). Melatonin ameliorates cognitive impairment induced by sleep deprivation in rats: role of oxidative stress, BDNF and CaMKII. *Behav Brain Res., 1*(256), 72-81.

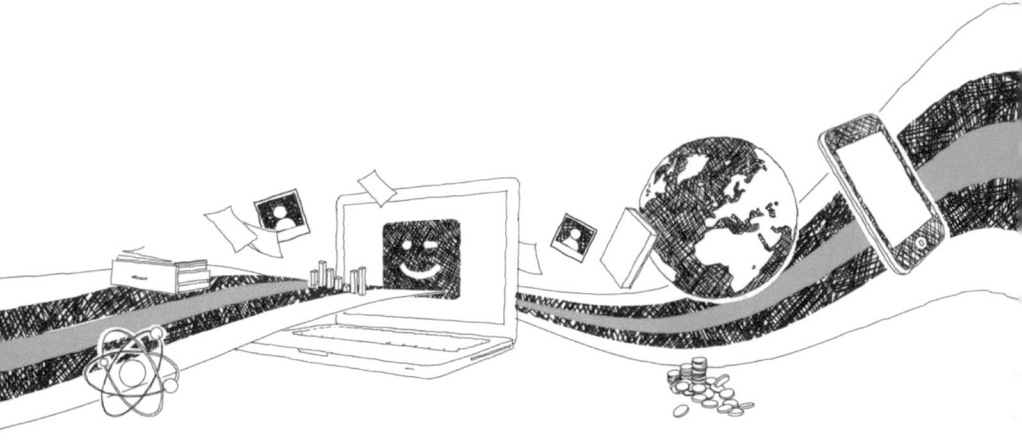
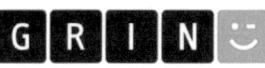